64 Habits

for a

Healthy Life

A guide on how to live a healthier
more rewarding life

ROXANNE MARTIN

Table of content

INTRODUCTION

A healthy lifestyle is a way of living that lowers the risk of being seriously ill or dying early. Not all diseases are preventable, but a large proportion of deaths, particularly those from coronary heart disease and lung cancer, can be avoided. Scientific studies have identified certain types of behavior that contributes to the development of no communicable diseases and early death. Health is not just about avoiding disease. It is also about physical, mental and social well-being. When a healthy lifestyle is adopted, a more positive role model is provided for other people in the family, particularly children.

The key to better health is to make small changes you can gradually build into your daily routine — and stick with them. You don't need to make all these changes at once. First, look at the ideas listed here, and give yourself a gold star for everything you're already doing. Then choose just one or two healthy changes you're ready to make right now. When they become habits, you'll be ready to add in another one.

WHAT MAKES A HABIT SO POWERFUL?

Daily habits are powerful – perhaps more powerful than you realize.

We tend to place a lot of emphasis on the big decisions in life such as whether or not we get married or where we go to college. These are important; but we tend to discount daily habits, even though those small, seemingly insignificant routines are just as influential.

Consider the following habits...

What you eat for breakfast today may not seem to matter, but what you eat for breakfast every day may determine whether you are obese or slender, healthy or unhealthy. It may determine whether you live to 100 or die of a heart attack at age 50.

How much sleep you get today may not seem to matter, but your overall sleep quality may affect your mental health to the point where it affects your ability to hold a job, advance professionally, interact respectfully with others and even maintain a love relationship with a partner.

Your silence in a meeting at work today may not seem to influence your career path, but a lifetime of hesitancy and self-doubt may cost you hundreds of thousands of dollars in potential income.

A way of living that LOWERS THE RISK of being seriously ill or dying early. Not all illness and disease is preventable;

however, a large proportion of deaths, particularly those from coronary heart disease and lung cancer, can be avoided. Scientific studies have identified certain types of behavior that contribute to serious illness and early death. This booklet aims at helping you to change your behavior and IMPROVE YOUR HEALTH so that you and your family live healthier longer lives.

Why Focus on Developing Daily Habits?

A habit is a regular tendency or practice. It's something you do almost without thinking. In some cases, our habits even come to define us as people.

You may consider yourself an "early riser," but you're just in the habit of getting up early. You may think of your neighbor as a runner, but she's just in the habit of running.

When we get in the habit of doing something, it no longer takes the tremendous amount of effort a new activity requires. That's why you'll find yourself swinging through the Dunkin' Donuts drive through instead of searching for a healthier breakfast option (familiar is comforting, it requires less thought, it feels right – all because it's a habit.)

Your habits also relate to why you'll put up with unpleasant tasks at work (you're in the habit of just saying yes, and it would take more effort to negotiate) or settle for boring instead of seeking adventure.

We're creatures of habit, and the many daily habits we have become accustomed to are the very fabric of our lives.

Healthy Habits? Healthy You!

I've found that creating healthy habits can improve your quality of life significantly. That's why I'm going to share the most powerful positive habits I've found for improving your life.

As you tackle this book, I encourage you to take steps to break these habits into something more manageable.

For your convenience, I've divided the book into three sections, offering positive daily habits for the following aspects of your life:

- Work
- Sleep
- Health

Each of the habits presented in this book is completely doable. Establishing the new habit will not be difficult. Your goal is to focus on the new practice until it replaces your old habits. That's the beauty of daily habits: they are small enough to be easy, yet the result of establishing that new habit is exponential in scope.

For optimal results, read the entire book at once, and then tackle this book in one of the following ways:

- Commit to establishing new habits in just one area of your life, concentrating on one segment of the book until you feel you have made adequate progress
- Choose one habit at a time until you've got that one habit down, and then add a new habit to your repertoire after that

- Choose your favorite habits out of the habits suggested, and tackle them one by one until you've established all your favorite new habits

Whatever way you choose to approach this challenge, I encourage you to take the time to enjoy the process. Improving your life is fun. It involves dreaming and assessing, growing and changing.

How do I know?

I'm certainly not perfect.

In fact, I'm still working on establishing some of the habits listed here in this book.

But I do know this: every positive habit I establish is one more step in the right direction, and I can feel the positive impact on my life overall. My wish for you is a similar experience as you enrich your life through the development of positive habits.

WORK HABITS THAT PAY DIVIDENDS

Many of us work more hours than we sleep in a day, and most of us spend far more time working than we spend on any other activity.

Your work experience impacts the rest of your life.

If you have a good day at work, you are more likely to come home refreshed and ready to dive into something engaging at home.

If you come home from work exhausted, frustrated or depressed by your job, you will be less likely to engage in fun activities at home. You might snap at your husband or wife, or be too tired to enjoy the kids. Your friends might call, hoping you'll be free to go out, but you won't have the energy to enjoy the leisure hours of your life.

Your working hours also impact your income potential, your satisfaction, and your career path.

That's why there are highly effective work habits that can transform your work experience, making you happier and more effective at your workplace.

1. Arrive Fifteen Minutes Before Necessary

One of the best ways to set yourself up for work success is to get to work before you need to be there.

If you are in the habit of scooting in just before your first meeting, you're probably dealing with at least one of the following:

- Anxiety over how your coworkers perceive you
- Speeding on the way to work
- Inability to smile and greet coworkers pleasantly
- Lack of planning time before you have to dive into actual work
- In a nutshell, unnecessary stress

Perhaps you're one of those rare birds who perform well under stress, but most of us flounder.

Coming to work late or barely on time puts you at risk for:

- A computer that won't start up right away, making you late
- A parking complication or other unforeseen troubles with transportation
- Realizing you didn't finish that report that is due first thing in the morning

If you always arrive early, you will build a cushion that will protect you from undue stress. It's the best way to arrive at work calm, positive, relaxed and guilt free.

To establish this habit, you will need to leave your house fifteen minutes earlier than you usually do. By doing this, you'll improve your performance and protect your mental health, all the while bolstering your reputation around the office.

2. Choose One Way to Excel Each Day

It's easy to get bogged down at work, forgetting your end goal. Perhaps you took on a job as a software engineer, and you love programming, but you hate all those meetings you must attend before you get to program. It's easy to get discouraged and lose enthusiasm.

When you let one piece of the job drag you down, it affects your overall performance. This can negatively impact your ability to grow your career.

One habit you can cultivate that will combat this negative spiral is this:

Choose one way to excel at your job on a daily basis. Link this one effort to something bigger than the job you already have.

For example, let's say you are a graphic designer. You don't really like the project you're currently on, and the meetings are a drag. However, you hope to start your graphic design firm someday (or even to just contract on your own, working independently.)

What will you need to get a new job or to land clients when you start your own firm? A great portfolio, right?

Choose to excel in your actual graphic design work each day, even if the actual project is boring (like a logo for a plumber), keeping in mind that you can use the project as part of your portfolio if you do a good enough job.

Grit your teeth and get through the meetings required, but pour yourself into the actual design work, creating something you are truly proud of.

Start your day with the daily habit of choosing one piece to excel in, and you'll build something impressive over time, regardless of how wonderful or awful your current position is.

3. Race Against Yourself

It's easy to get distracted and derailed. You get emails, text messages, and instant messages all day long. You go online to research something for work, and some stupid Yahoo article title catches your eye. Perhaps you work from home where you have a laundry list of distractions that call your name all day long.

You can beat the distraction demons by setting small goals for yourself and then race against the clock to beat your estimated time frame.

Make a habit of setting a goal regarding how much you want to get done each day. Then divide the work into small segments anywhere from 30 minutes to an hour's worth of work at a time. Then set a timer for yourself and race against yourself to see if you really can achieve your goals.

By working in short bursts and setting small goals, you'll find your productivity will far exceed whatever you'd meander through is you proceed without deadlines or goals.

4. Incorporate Stress Management Into Your Work Day

Do you work in a stressful environment?

That's why you'll want to incorporate a simple form of stress management into your workday.

One highly effective way to manage stress is to breathe deeply for five minutes.

When a meeting is getting stressful or a day feels harried, excuse yourself to your office, cubicle, restroom or car. Then close your eyes and focus on nothing but your breathing. Set a timer for five minutes and refuse to think about anything else besides how marvelous it feels to breathe in and out.

5. Network

Whether you love your current job or hate it, networking is always a wise move.

Why?

It's close to impossible to know what your work situation will be five years from now, even if you're in a stable field, and knowing someone who knows someone is the best way to get a new job or line up a new client.

How do establish a habit of networking?

First off, always bring business cards with you wherever you go, and hand them out freely. Be sure to keep up with contacts from time to time, connecting on social networks like LinkedIn, so you have a way to get back in touch later on.

6. Play to Your Strengths

We all have strengths and weaknesses.

You also have strengths and weaknesses. If you make a habit of using your strengths but delegating your weaknesses to someone else, you will excel in your career.

This is easier to do if you run your own business than if you work a 9-5 job for the man, but you really can make this shift in most work environments.

Collaborate with coworkers on projects or talk to your manager about taking on more work that suits your strengths and shifting assignments that trip you up to someone who is more competent in that area. If your boss is unyielding, look for a new position somewhere that will allow you to use your strengths.

7. Take a Real Lunch Break

If you've been eating at your desk, you're cheating yourself—and your co-workers

Work study experts conclude that taking a real lunch break will improve your productivity and prevent job burnout. That means you should at least leave your desk and enjoy a meal where you're not engaged in work activities.

Better yet, walk to a nearby lunch destination. Even if you just walk two blocks to a local restaurant and walk back again, this will help you manage work stress. Moving your body, getting outside in the sun, and getting out of the office all works together to relieve stress and rejuvenate your spirit.

8. Always Look for Intrinsic Rewards

You might have a boring job right now. If this is the case, you can either let the job rot your brain out, or you can take control of your destiny. One way you can do this is to daily find an intrinsic reward that has been hidden in your work.

What does this mean practically?

Each day you need to find one thing that makes you feel good about doing your job. Maybe it's knowing you helped someone figure out how to use their bank account or that you felt fabulous about getting through that huge stack of mortgage papers that needed to get evaluated and processed.

 Look for rewards that truly make you proud of yourself. Then write down your one accomplishment each day. Believe it or not, this will help you avoid burnout at your job.

9. Add a "Wake Up" Routine in the Afternoon

Perk up in the afternoon (your body automatically enters an energy slump somewhere between one and three every afternoon) by using a natural stimulant. A lot of people enjoy caffeine in its various forms, but some people find an afternoon cup of coffee or soda will interfere with sleep at night. Try the following and see which you can build into your daily afternoon routine:

- Put a drop of peppermint essential oil under your nose (you will feel more mentally alert).
- Drink a cup of yerba mate tea (this tea contains a mellow stimulant that acts like caffeine but will not make you jittery or interfere with sleep).
- Do jumping jacks or run in place for three minutes.
- Stretch for three minutes (sun salutations are perfect, but any stretch will do).

By incorporating an invigorating practice into your afternoon routine, you will be more productive and enthusiastic at a time of day when you might otherwise be sleepy and unmotivated.

10. Sandbag When Estimating

It's important to be known at work as reliable and dependable. That's why you should get in the habit of sandbagging, which means padding any estimate on time, money or resources needed to complete a project.

It's tempting to say you can get a job quickly, but it's better to prepare for obstacles. People who routinely come in under budget and on time are going to be trusted and respected more than the people who give optimistic projections and then fall short.

Make it a habit of asking for more time, money and resources than you think you will need.

11. Make Yourself Known

You probably don't have problems doing this if you are an extrovert, but many introverts find themselves quietly doing their duties—and then being passed over at bonus time.

Make it a habit of speaking up at least once in every meeting.

Instead of zoning out in meetings and biding your time until you can get to the "real work," look for ways to add insight and value vocally.

This is especially important if you work remotely. If people don't know who you are and what you contribute, you will be the first one on the chopping block when it comes time for layoffs.

If you happen to be a talker, you may wish to scale back how much you contribute, focusing instead on contributing only valuable input. You don't want to be known as a boorish person who monopolizes meetings. Instead, you need to stand out for useful, helpful contributions.

12. Document Everything Important

While you'd like to believe your manager, co-workers and clients will always remember agreements and negotiations the same way you remember them; it's very likely you will encounter disagreements at one point or another.

To keep communication clear and to prevent misunderstandings, you will want to make a habit of documenting the following:

- Project specifications and deadlines
- Any discussion of pay rates raises or bonuses
- Expectations expressed in meetings
- Customer or client issues
- Problems with coworkers

Get everything in writing. You can do this by documenting through an email or notes on your computer. If you are documenting sensitive information, password protect your document so coworkers can't possibly get access to it without your permission.

Then, if someone later remembers a bonus discussion differently than you do, you can check that email or note to yourself and bring the documentation to the table for discussion.

13. Avoid Gossiping

Does your coworker drive you batty?

If it hasn't happened to you yet, it probably will someday. It's tempted to gossip with your friends about "Loud Larry" or "Mustache Mary," but you'd better think before you start sharing such thoughts with anyone even vaguely related to your career.

It's best to assume that you will have to work with this person again someday, and the next time around, Loud Larry might be your boss. Mustache Mary might be on the review board evaluating your resume for a new position.

Treat co-workers with respect and keep personal grudges out of the work arena altogether.

14. Find a Way to Laugh

Work-related stress can do more than get you down. It can also interfere with progress and cooperation in the workplace.

One of the best ways to diffuse stress and restore morale is through laughter.

In fact, corporate human resource divisions are beginning to recognize the value of programs like laughter therapy, laughter yoga classes, and laughter clubs.

Scientists like Charles Schaefer, a psychology professor at Fairleigh Dickinson University, have discovered that even forced laughter can cause physiological changes that help people feel better.

Your company may not be ready to hold laughter yoga sessions, but you can lighten the mood during meetings and improve overall morale by getting in touch with your internal stand-up comedian. Crack a joke when appropriate, and let it rip with a couple of close coworkers over lunch. A good laugh will help you work better and live better.

15. Ask For What You Need

Have you complained to your friends about something at work? Perhaps you're sick of the snarky way your coworker talks to you, or you feel there's never enough time to complete projects?

These complaints, if gone unrecognized, are exactly the sorts of things that end up decreasing work productivity and later resulting in termination or you deciding the job isn't worth it. In fact, a study published in Forbes lists lack or respect and lack of work-life balance as two of the top five reasons people quit their jobs.

Talk to management about complaints, explaining exactly what you need and why you need it. You'll be surprised at how willing most companies are to provide exactly what you need – if you ask clearly and directly, without accusing anyone of wrongdoing.

Silently holding onto resentment about unmet (and often unexpressed) needs will often build to the point where you will feel the need to quit. That's why it's better to ask to be moved to a new group or express your need for more time to finish projects than just silently seethe at your desk.

16. Leverage the 80/20 Rule

You've heard the theory that most people get 80 percent of the work done in 20 percent of the time they spend on a project, haven't you?

That's because we're not designed to work at full efficiency at all times. We have productive times of day and unproductive times, productive environments and unproductive environments.

The key is this: Make sure you are working on the most important projects during your most productive space of each day.

What does that mean practically?

Early birds like me should prioritize our most important work for the early morning, leaving less important work for the afternoon. Those who peak in solitude should save their most important work for times when they work alone.

Those who work best as a group should schedule important tasks to be tackled with coworkers. That may mean you have to alter your schedule or talk to your manager. Maybe you want to come to work an hour early or stay after everyone else leaves at night. Maybe you'll want to ask if you can work from home one day a week or collaborate with coworkers on specific projects.

Find your sweet spot, and then make sure you're tackling the most important tasks in the best way and time.

SLEEP HABITS

Believe it or not, not everyone needs the much-prescribed eight hours of sleep everyone talks about. In fact, sleep needs range from a mere five and a half to a mighty ten hours per night. That means you need to figure out how much sleep you need, and then figure out how to get it.

The following habits will help you get your much-needed sleep, which will help you function better in the rest of your life.

17. Plan for Adequate Sleep

First off, find out how much sleep you need for optimal functionality. You will want to set aside a week for this experiment, allowing yourself to go to bed whenever feels natural and then wake up whenever feels natural. Record your number of hours of sleep you got each night, and make a note of how you felt each day afterward. For those first couple nights, you may be catching up on sleep if you were sleep deprived, but you should settle into a routine by the end of the week.

Now that you know how much sleep you need, you will need to block out that much time plus one hour each night.

Why the extra hour? Because you'll want to start incorporating the habits listed below into that hour just before you turn out the lights. Schedule your sleep time as if it were an appointment, and treat it as such.

After all, it's an appointment with restoration and rejuvenation, something we all need.

18. Reserve the Bedroom for Sleep-Related Activities

Many of us use our bedrooms as an extra living room or craft room. Maybe you head to the bedroom right after dinner to settle in for a board game with your child or to watch TV with your partner.

If you've been using your bedroom as a living room, you'll probably want to move those evening activities to another part of the house.

Why?

Making a psychological separation between your bedroom (where you sleep) and activity rooms (kitchen, TV room, and office) will help you associate your bedroom with sleeping. This will help you leave your anxieties from work and bill-related worries in the office, electronic stimulation in the TV room and stress of household chores in the kitchen.

Many people find that making this distinction frees them up for much sounder sleep.

19. Don't Exercise Right Before Bedtime

If you can't exercise before work or over your lunch break, you will want to exercise right after work, ending your exercise session at least two hours before you plan on retiring for the evening.

Why?

Your body will remain revved up and energized for about two hours after you exercise (especially if you exercise vigorously), making it hard for you to fall asleep.

However, a vigorous workout, followed up by a bath or shower and two hours of relaxation time, will result in sound, peaceful sleep that will both nourish you and help your body recuperate.

20. Stop Using Electronics Right Before Bedtime

Internet surfers, gamers, and television junkies be warned! All that time spent on electronics can get you so jazzed up inside that you can't sleep well. The visual stimulation you experience when using electronics creates a buzz inside your head that lingers, interfering with sleep.

What should you do for that last hour before bed? Try reading, journaling or doing a puzzle instead.

All of these recommended activities are calming and will help you fall asleep easier.

21. Drink the Right "Sleepy Time" Drink

That glass of wine might make you feel sleepy, but cut yourself off after one glass or you'll sleep less soundly than if you abstained altogether.

Looking for the best sleepy-time beverages? Valerian or chamomile tea work wonders, as does the infamous warm milk. Some people can handle caffeine even right before bed, but most people need to stop drinking caffeine around four in the afternoon if they want to sleep soundly.

That means you need to avoid coffee, hot chocolate, and even decaffeinated green or black tea – they still contain traces of caffeine. Go for herbal teas instead.

22. Purge All Anxious Thoughts

Most of us encounter some stress each day. It might be positive stress (you're in love, you finished a big project at work) or it might be negative stress (you missed a deadline at work, your neighbor snarked at you about the dog barking, you found out your son has a D in Social Studies.)

Perhaps you are worried about potential problems (what if your daughter doesn't catch the bus tomorrow and you end up late for that client meeting because you have to drive her to school; what if your boyfriend didn't text back because he's thinking about breaking up.)

Whatever the case may be, most of us end the day with a stockpile of emotions and thoughts raging through our heads. We need a way to empty out all those thoughts, put them into perspective and then lock them away for the night so we can get some decent shut-eye. That's why you'll want to make a habit of purging all anxious thoughts at least an hour before you go to bed.

The following are very effective purging practices:

- Talk to a friend
- Write in a journal

- Participate in an online advice forum
- Write your concerns on Post It notes and then put them in a drawer
- Plan out your next day to avoid surprises and to help yourself feel in control

After you've dumped out your concerns, you'll want to relax for that last remaining hour, doing something that distracts you from anxiety and helps you settle into a content feeling of "everything will be okay."

23. Meditate or Pray for Ten Minutes

Set a timer, shut your eyes, sit in a comfortable position and surrender your worries to a higher being. Even if you're not religious, ten minutes of meditation (repeating a mantra or focusing on your breathing) will help you relax enough to sleep soundly.

24. Engage in a Flow Activity

"Flow" activities are repetitive activities that you can do without concentrating. Psychologists have found that such activities calm your nervous system and will help you feel content, grounded and secure – all of which will help you sleep better.

Make it a habit to daily engage in a flow activity such as the following:

Painting, knitting, woodworking, cleaning or folding laundry. Relax into the activity and allow your mind to wander wherever it may. You will subconsciously deal with stress from the day, explore creative ideas, and end the flow activity feeling more relaxed. You'll sleep better because of it.

25. Adjust the Lights

Replace bright light bulbs with softer light in your bedroom, signaling to your body that it is time to go to sleep.

We were designed to be light sensitive so we would wake with the morning sun and go to bed soon after the sunset. Use low wattage, golden light bulbs (never those harsh white fluorescent bulbs) in your bedroom. Better yet, light candles. You'll be sleepy before you know it!

26. Turn Up the Music

Of course, I'm not talking about rock or screaming heavy metal music. Calming sound cues help us relax. Scientists believe this is linked to the constant sounds we heard while in the womb, lulling us to sleep.

As adults, calming musical rhythms such as the sound of waves, wind, rain or soothing music signals to our body that it's time to sleep.

27. Turn Down the Room Temperature

Even if you like to be warm, you'll sleep better in a cool room. This is because your body's core temperature lowers as you go to sleep, rising when it gets closer to your time to wake back up.

Lower the thermostat by a couple of degrees and pile on the blankets.

The combination of cool room temperature and snuggly, heavy blankets on you will make you feel warm, cozy and secure – the perfect combination for a perfect night of sleep.

28. Cover All Sources of Light

Ever get the feeling a dozen eyes are staring at you as you lie in bed?

Those would be the many LED lights you have in your room. Cover LED lights or block them from your view.

Most people sleep best in complete darkness, so you'll want to move computers and extra electronics out of the bedroom so you can make it as dark as possible.

29. Indulge a Calming Experience

Take a hot bath, give your partner a massage (and then receive one), engage in sex or stretch your muscles for a good 20-30 minutes in that hour before you go to sleep. All of these activities involve your senses and promote genuine relaxation.

30. Sniff Deeply

Your massage therapist isn't using lavender essential oil just because he likes floral scents. Scientific tests have proven that lavender and geranium scents (essential oils, not artificial synthetic scents) lower blood pressure and slow your heart rate. Invest in an essential oil diffuser for your bedroom and diffuse a couple of drops of a calming essential oil each night right before bed for a peaceful night of sleep.

31. Get Help with Your Sleep

Does your partner like to stay up later than you? Ask him or her to cuddle with you for five minutes, even if he or she is going to get back up again. Why?

Cuddling helps lower our blood pressure and heart rates, and it helps us feel secure so that we can drift off to sleep.

We are designed to want to have something living close to us when we fall asleep. That's why cuddling with a child, pet or partner will all help you fall asleep. Listen to your snuggle buddy's breathing and pay attention to how good it feels to have a warm body up against you. You'll be out in no time.

32. Knock Yourself Out

If you've tried all of the habits mentioned above and still can't sleep, you'll want to try taking melatonin, a natural supplement that your body already produces. Melatonin works in conjunction with light exposure. Our body produces melatonin each night after the sun sets, signaling to our body that its time to rest.

Many over the counter sleep aids are simply decongestants repackaged, and most of them leave you groggy the next morning. You can take three to five milligrams of melatonin right before bed and still feel great in the morning.

Melatonin is non-habit-forming, but it's a fine habit to establish if you need help falling asleep but don't want to be foggy-headed the next morning.

HABITS FOR A HAPPIER AND HEALTHIER LIFE

34. Don't overeat

If you want to live to 100, leaving a little bit of food on your plate may be a good idea. Author Dan Buettner, who studies durability around the world, found that the oldest Japanese people stop eating when they are feeling only about 80% full.

St. Louis University researchers have confirmed that eating less helps you age slower. They found that limiting calories lowered production of T3, a thyroid hormone that slows metabolism—and speeds up the aging process.

35. Turn off the TV

Too much time in front of the TV can take a serious toll on your health. People who watched four or more hours a day were 46% more likely to die from any cause than people who watched less than two hours a day.

Even cutting back a little can help; each additional hour you watch increases your overall risk of dying by 11% and dying from heart disease by 18%.

36. Stay out of the sun

Avoiding too much sun can take off skin cancer, and it can also keep you looking young by preventing wrinkles, fine lines, and saggy skin.

It's never too early or too late to add sunscreen to your daily skin-care regimen (look for an SPF of 30 or higher). And don't focus only on your face. Sun damage spots and splotches on your chest and neck will also make you appear older.

37. Reach out

You're at greater risk of heart disease without a strong network of friends and family. Loneliness can cause inflammation, and in otherwise healthy people it can be just as dangerous as having high cholesterol or even smoking.

Loneliness seems to pose the greatest risk for elderly people, who are also prone to depression.

38. Drink in moderation

Women who have two or more drinks a day and men who have three or more may run into detrimental effects ranging from weight gain to relationship problems. But in smaller quantities, alcohol can be good for you.

A 2010 study in the Journal of the American College of Cardiology linked light drinking (one drink a day for women and two for men) to significant heart benefits.

39. Eat fruits and vegetables

Getting fewer than three servings of fruits and vegetables a day can harm your health. Nutritional powerhouses filled with fiber and vitamins, fruits and veggies can lower your risk of heart disease by 76% and may even play a role in decreasing your risk of breast cancer.

As an added bonus, the inflammation-fighting and circulation-boosting powers of the antioxidants in fruits and veggies can banish wrinkles.

40. Don't smoke

Quitting smoking is perhaps the single most important thing you can do for your health and your life span. It is said that women who quit smoking by age 35 add roughly six to eight years to their lives.

It's never too late to kick the habit. Quitting can slow disease and increase survival odds even in smokers who have already caused significant damage to their lungs, like those with early lung cancer.

41. Focus on fitness

Daily exercise may be the closest thing we have to a fountain of youth. A 2008 study found that regular high-intensity exercise (such as running) can add up to four years to your life, which isn't surprising given the positive effects working out has on your heart, mind, and metabolism.

Even moderate exercise a quick, 30-minute walk each day,

for example can lower your risk of heart problems.

42. Live a balanced lifestyle

It is hard to try and have time to do everything that is important to you, but it is important that you do try. The best thing to achieving this is to get organized and work out what your goals are and what you want to achieve.

43. Know yourself and take corrective action

If you know that you're a workaholic, get a diary, find a hobby and make time for yourself and for you to enjoy yourself. If you don't exactly have the best diet in the world, try to start eating healthily and take vitamins and supplements. If you are struggling with your weight, look for healthy recipes and natural tips to assist and support you in your weight loss... and make sure you follow them. Critically evaluating yourself is important and crucial in ensuring that any lifestyle change is a true lifestyle change that will last your lifetime. Understand your weakness and don't be afraid to change and correct them. You will feel much more fulfilled when you do succeed and you'll also become a better and healthier person with each passing day.

44. Stop Using Toxic Chemicals In Your Home

Start reading labels and becoming familiar with what is in your cleaning products; most of them contain really dangerous substances that you probably wouldn't choose to use in your home. Be on the look-out for ingredients like formaldehyde, phenol and triclosan, and stay as far away from them as possible.

45. Recycle

Instead of filling landfills with waste, try and recycle paper, glass, tin and plastic. Try and find ways to reuse your own waste and make a concerted effort to purchase products that use biodegradable packaging. This is a great long term strategy for us all to live longer, with less pollution.

46. Go Organic

Start buying organic products that have not been grown with chemicals or pesticides, produced by companies that are making an effort to reduce their carbon footprint. Your family will be healthier for it and it will take less of a toll on the environment. Start eating free range eggs and meat, and consider going a day where you do not eat meat, as animals reared for food are some of the biggest sources of methane gas on the planet.

There are a number of different things that determines how long we will live and the fact still remains that luck seems to play an incredibly large role, as does heredity. Fortunately there are three other factors that we can control ourselves that seem to have a large impact on how long we will live and its those exact things that I'm going to talk about in this article today.

The first thing is healthful lifestyle, which isn't a huge stretch of the imagination. If you eat a good diet and get regular exercise, and don't really do anything else at all, you can generally expect to live to around 80 years old or more

The second thing deals with nutritional supplements. Certain research has showed in the last few years that people who consume the optimum level of certain key vitamins and minerals can often expect to live as much as 15 years longer than normal people.

The third thing is hormone therapy. Certain studies have shown that animals who are given certain hormones as well as other drugs are able to live 20% to 35% longer than animals who were not given the same hormones and other drugs. Basically, in human terms that comes to about 120 years of age which is not too shabby.

Some of the different hormone therapies that may or may not help include testosterone replacement therapy which boosts sex drive and strengthens bones in men and women, human growth hormone therapy which has been shown to smooth wrinkles and strengthen a weak libido, melatonin therapy which has been shown to extend the lifespan of mice by up to 25% and DHEA therapy which can boost immune functions and may fight cancer as well as heart disease and other diseases as well. Of course, any type of hormone therapy should be massively supervised by a doctor or not done at all.

Yes, these three things that I just mentioned are rather broad and not incredibly specific but they still give you a pretty good idea of what it takes to live longer today. Basically it comes down to the same formula you know in your heart already; eat a well-balanced diet stay away from junk food and alcohol, exercise regularly, take your vitamins and minerals, keep an eye on less traditional methods such as hormone therapy and you should live a long healthful life.

Antiaging health is a full body experience that must be taken seriously. The internal mechanisms, including the psychological aspects, must also be taken into account. "Feeling young" is important to antiaging health. It all comes down to mind over matter. If you have the desire to work out the exercise will become easier.

Many people ignore the realities of aging until it is too late. Many more look for quick fixes and try to beat aging by improving the look and feel of their skin. Those who adhere to the natural anti aging school of thought, however, tend to have a more well-rounded approach to aging and are more apt to defeat the signs of aging in a reasonable way.

For all age groups an active mental and physical approach to life will improve our feel good factor, just get off your backside and do something. Virtually anything is better than doing nothing! Even if you want an unhealthy late night meal, don't ring up the delivered at home service, or get in your car to pick one up from the takeaway, go and walk to pick it up. Or even better still get go hungry and look forward to a great healthy breakfast in a few hours time.

HABITS FOR A HEALTHY MIND

Happiness is one of the most sought-after goals in life, yet for many it seems to be mysterious. It's easy to delude ourselves into thinking, "When I just have that nice house and new car, then I can be happy." But in reality, happiness is available to all of us, right now. A big house or a new car won't actually make you happier; it's the simple joys in life that bring true happiness.

47. Do What You Love

If your passion is playing soccer, writing poems, or teaching children how to swim, make time to do it. You'll find that when you're doing what you love, you're filled with joy. How much better does that sound than forcing yourself do something you don't like?

48. Help Others

Sometimes after we've achieved our own personal goals, we still feel empty inside because we haven't made a meaningful contribution to someone else's life. When we volunteer or help others, it feels good to just be of service to someone else. The impact we make feels fulfilling and is a big potential source for our own happiness.

49. Be Thankful

When you think of all the things that you have to be grateful for, you realize how blessed you already are. Without even realizing it, we take our basic necessities for granted like a roof over your head and plenty of food to eat. By appreciating the things that you already have, you'll begin to feel happier and healthier in your life.

Share With Others

When we share our thoughts, our time, and our abilities with others we feel better for it. A life lived without sharing can become lonely. When you share with others, they'll feel great towards you and help you to feel more joy in your own life.

50. Smile More

Practice smiling more and see how it affects you internally, as well as those around you. You can always afford to give a smile. Smiling can make you happier even if you have to force it, you'll still feel better.

51. Exercise

When was the last time you went to the gym or worked out? Exercise reduces stress and releases endorphins, also known as a "runner's high." Playing sports is a fun way to exercise as well, whether it's kicking around a soccer ball or shooting hoops.

52. Get a Life Coach

A life coach will help you to evaluate your life and why you're not feeling happy in it. Maybe you're holding limiting beliefs or you have an emotional block without realizing it. By speaking to a life coach, you can uncover why you're actually unhappy and what you can do to feel better.

Find Ways to Manage Stress

Don't let stress rob you of your birthright to be happy. You deserve to be happy, and it wouldn't be right to let stress get in the way. Practices such as meditation can help you to manage stress better and feel great.

53. Forgive and Forget

Holding a grudge will harm you more than the person you're holding it against. Ask yourself, "What would it take for me to let go of the past?" and notice how you feel when you let go of your anger for a few seconds. Focus instead on a bright future and you'll feel better for it.

54. Be Yourself

As Steve Jobs said, "Your time is limited, so don't waste it living someone else's life." Accept who you are, just be yourself, and you'll feel a world of difference.

55. Spend Time With Your Loved Ones

There's no replacement for spending quality time with your loved ones. We're social beings, even if you're an introvert or a loner. People love spending time with their friends and family for good conversation, bonding, and some laughs. Life's too short to live it completely alone.

56. Do Away With Negative Thinking

You already know that negative thinking will bring you down. So how do you stop it? Become more aware of it and try replacing your negative thoughts with some positive ones. Spend less time with negative people and more time with positive people.

57. Give More Gifts

You don't have to give expensive gifts; sometimes a poem, a quick note, or a thoughtful email will brighten someone else's day, and yours. Share what you can give to all the wonderful people in your life.

HABITS FOR A HEALTHY BODY

Protecting your body could start with buckling your seatbelt when in a vehicle, wearing a helmet when riding a bike or motorcycle, using elbow and kneepads when skateboarding, and so forth.

Protecting your body could include using sunscreen and protection from bug bites.

The harmful effects of stress can wreak havoc on your body as you age. Fight back by protecting your most vulnerable organs. Keep your eyes, skin and liver healthy and vital with these three powerful nutrients.

Lutein for Your Eyes

As you get older, your eyes become vulnerable to macular degeneration, a disease that can severely damage your vision. Lutein protects your eyes from the oxidative stress and free radical damage that could harm your eyesight. Look for at least 8 mg in your multivitamin, or you can get your daily dose from foods like kale, papaya and eggs.

Zinc for Your Skin

This nutrient acts as a 24-hour on-call skin mechanic. Zinc repairs the wear and tear caused by stressors to your skin. It works to heal tissue by stimulating cell growth and regeneration. Look for zinc in supplement form. Try a dose of at least 8 mg in your multivitamin. Zinc is also found in many foods: Swiss and cheddar cheese, yogurt, baked beans, oysters, crab and lobster.

Glucosinolates for Your Liver

Your liver is responsible for detoxifying your body. Glucosinolates can help protect your liver by regulating the enzymes that assist in the detoxification process. The best way to get this important phytonutrient is through food sources like collard greens, Brussels sprouts and cauliflower.

Habits that make you age faster and look older

Smoking

It is a known fact that smoking harms your health in many ways. But smoking can also accelerate the aging process of your skin. The harmful chemicals in cigarette smoke chronically deprive your skin cells of oxygen, which can lead to pale, uneven coloring. It even triggers the breakdown of collagen and can cause loose, saggy skin. In fact, the whole process of smoking can cause deep wrinkles around the mouth.

Those who are more concerned about their appearance should try to stop smoking. Whether you smoke or you spend time with a smoker, cigarette smoke is bad for your skin. By quitting smoking and avoiding secondhand smoke, you can restore your skin's health. Quitting smoking improves skin conditions and, above all, skin-aging effects.

Drinking in Excess

Alcohol is a natural diuretic, so when you drink in excess it causes dehydration. Dehydration depletes the natural moisture from your skin, which automatically makes you look older than your age.

Excess alcohol intake causes a depletion of healthy nutrients in your body, particularly vitamins A and C. These antioxidant vitamins are essentail for maintaining vibrant and supple skin. Plus, excessive alcohol intake is one of the triggers for rosacea outbreaks. High alcohol intake is even associated with skin cancer.

Higher current alcohol intake, higher lifetime alcohol intake and even a higher preference for white wine or liquor were associated with increased risk of melanoma and non-melanoma skin cancer.

This does not mean that you cannot enjoy having a drink at all. Just drink in moderation or occasionally. According to the American Heart Association, men should limit themselves to 1 to 2 drinks a day, and women to 1 drink a day (1 drink is 12 ounces of beer or 4 ounces of wine).

Holding Grudges

Forgiveness is something most of us believe in, but we don't always practice it. Holding grudges against any person or situation is not good for your health as well as appearance.

If you are not able to forgive, you are adding more stress to your life, which boosts your level of the hormone cortisol. Cortisol leads to weight gain, high blood pressure and high blood sugar. Stress even leads to more frowning, one of the key causes of wrinkles on the forehead. Stress is a common cause of a lot many health problems and also contributes to aging. Do not allow an old grudge to sap your youthfulness. Practice forgiveness and experience better mental and physical well-being.

Sun Exposure

No matter how amazing the sun feels on your body, regular and prolonged exposure to sunrays is one of the worst things you can do for your skin. Long-term exposure to harmful ultraviolet (UV) rays of the sun weakens your skin cells and blood vessels, which causes a tanned, leathery-looking skin. It even leads to pigmentation, reduced skin elasticity and a degradation of skin texture. Also, the risk of skin cancer is significantly higher due to sun exposure. Freckles can turn into brown sun spots, the skin takes on a dry, leathery appearance, and wrinkles and sagging increase. Before going out in the sun, protect your skin by wear a hat, covering up with clothing and using sunscreen that is broad-spectrum, SPF 30 (or higher). You should apply sunscreen throughout the year. If you like a tanned look, apply a self-tanner rather than soaking up the sunrays. If you are worried about sun-damaged skin, consult a doctor to reduce existing damage.

Too Little Sleep

Just one night of bad sleep can make you look and feel tired. It can even lead to dark circles and bags under your eyes. Now, imagine what lack of sleep for days can do to your skin appearance. Sleep deprivation can cause skin damage in several ways. First of all, it can increase your cortisol level, which in turn can worsen inflammatory conditions. Secondly, it can cause poor collagen formation, which leads to skin aging. Poor sleepers had increased signs of skin aging and slower recovery from several environmental stressors, such as disruption of the skin barrier or UV radiation. Staying up late can be fun, but burning the midnight oil can make you look older as you age. To enjoy beautiful and flawless skin, make sleep a priority and try to get between 7 and 9 hours of sleep per night. But avoid sleeping too long on one side of your face, as it can cause wrinkles and sleep lines. Also, use a satin pillow case to avoid fine lines and wrinkles.

Feeding Your Sweet Tooth

A sugar-packed diet can take a toll on your waistline and weight. It can even speed up the skin-aging process. It can make your skin dull and wrinkled. This happens due to the process known as "glycation", in which sugar attaches to and damages proteins like collagen and elastin. These proteins are needed to keep skin smooth and flexible. In fact, drinking sugary sodas can lead to obesity, diabetes and heart attacks and may also speed up your body's aging process. Removing sugar from your diet is not easy if you have a sweet tooth. But you can definitely try to avoid processed sugar and opt for natural fruits to satisfy your cravings for sweets. You can even opt for dark chocolate, which is good for your health due to its high antioxidant content.

Spending Too Much Time On The Couch

Instead of being a couch potato and increasing your risk of obesity and other health problems, make exercise a part of your daily life. Exercise helps tone your muscles and gets your blood flowing so that your skin gets all the necessary nutrients. This has a regenerating effect on the skin. Plus, exercise provides you with lots of energy that helps you look and feel younger, at any age. Exercise even staves off heart disease, keeps stress at bay, fights brain fog, reduces inflammation, and prevents Type 2 diabetes and other chronic conditions that crop up with age. Take a break from your sedentary lifestyle and get moving. The American College of Sports Medicine recommends 30 minutes of moderate exercise most days of the week. Choose any activity you enjoy walking, swimming, cycling or dancing.

Eating Too Much Unhealthy Food

The food you eat has a direct impact on how your skin looks and the overall health of your body. If you wish to delay the aging process, you need to pay attention to your diet. Avoid inflammatory foods, such as vegetable oils, margarine, red meats, white bread and sugary, processed foods. These foods can cause inflammation in your body, which may hasten skin as well as overall aging. Eat foods rich in omega-3 fatty acids, such as flaxseeds, flaxseed oil, avocados, salmon and olive oil. These foods help fight inflammation to prevent chronic diseases and also keep your skin soft and supple. Eat plenty of fresh fruits and vegetables daily. Fruits and vegetables are abundant in zinc, selenium, vitamin C and beta-carotene, which aid the body's production of collagen. Also, eat protein-rich foods, as low protein intake can cause tears, wrinkles and cracks in the skin. Good sources of protein include eggs, lean meat, poultry and beans. Say no to junk food. The unhealthy levels of sodium, fat and cholesterol in these foods are not good for your skin as well as overall health. Lastly, do not ignore the importance of keeping your body hydrated. Drink an ample amount of water each day to prevent dehydration and to enjoy younger-looking skin.

You're glued to your desk all day.

Research shows that sitting all day can actually be deadly in the long run, in part because it increases the risk of cardiovascular disease. While you should always aim for a minimum of 30 minutes of moderate-to-vigorous exercise daily, if you reach that, but sit for the rest of the day, you're not necessarily lowering your risk for chronic disease.

HOW TO IMPROVE THE QUALITY OF LIFE

People have a huge impact on your life. You are the average of the five people you spend the most time with With this in mind, you should think about the people you're spending time with the same way you think about what you eat and how you're exercising.

Some people can be parasites. They suck out your happiness, energy and maybe some of your tangible resources as well. You can put spending time with them in the same category as eating nachos on the couch.

So what make someone a "good" person to spend time with? And what are the benefits of surrounding yourself with these people?

58. Surround yourself with good people

Good people aren't saints, or at least they don't have to be. They might spend their winter holidays helping starving children in Africa, or they may simply encourage you to hit the gym more. The good people you're looking for are positive, happy people that enrich your life. They can be: family members, friends, coworkers

Acquaintances that frequent the same coffee shop They are people that will inspire you to be a better person, provide you with motivation to achieve your goals, empower you to make the changes you need to succeed and cheer on your success. In the workplace, good people tend to be productive people. They're organized, create schedules they stick to and don't get easily distracted from the end goal. And all this help you be more productive!

It's important to note that "good" does not mean similar. Too much of the same thing can inhibit growth. You want to have diversity and healthy arguments. You should have an eagerness to soak up knowledge, and differing perspectives can help you with that. Think About the People You Spend the Most Time With Write down the qualities of the people you spend the most time with. Would you call them positive people? Happy? Now think of how they interact and affect you. Do they make you feel like you have what it takes to reach your goals? Do they support you? Do they make you feel attractive? Do you feel happy and energized after spending time with them? If you answered "yes" to these questions, you're probably already surrounded by the good people you need.

People are different. There are things that make you happy that might not make me happy. Your idea of support may differ from the next person's. The key is finding the people that are good for you.

So how do you do that?

Remember that like attracts like. You have to give off positive vibes and be confident. You also have to be yourself. This will lead you to the people that are right for you. You may also need to practice forgiveness. Resentment only breeds bitterness and unhappiness, and it's time to let the negativity go.

When you're surrounded by good people, you're surrounded by life. You'll be less stressed and find more joy in daily things. Today, make a commitment to start spending more time with the good people in your life.

Reasons It's Important to Surround Yourself with Positive People

Life is tough, and unfortunately there's no manual that comes with. Luckily, there are people that can help you through these events, no matter how intimidating the situation can be. These are the people worth having in your lives—because they bring positivity. Since people are a big part of our lives, it is crucial that you chose positive company and here are reasons why.

With positivity comes authenticity

Those with a positive outlook on life will look out for your wellbeing instead of trying to destroy it. They are looking to make a friend out of you- not an enemy.

A support system

Having a positive person in your life brings comfort. If you ever need a shoulder to cry on, you'll know who to turn to. Instead of keeping you down in the dumps they will try to uplift you, even if it's just lending an ear or lightening up the mood a bit.

Good vibes only

With these favorable people in your lives, good times are easier to have, even if it's just wanting to unwind for five minutes, because guess what? These type of people focus try to keep the mood flowing positively.

Drama free zone

No one likes drama. Those who practice positivity certainly don't have the time or energy for it. If you want to avoid these negative incidents then it's best you surround yourself with these type of people.

Motivation

Being around this sort of company will motivate you to stay clear of downward spirals and hopefully persuade you to make good and healthy decisions in life. Life is all about moving forward and it's imperative to be around those who help us navigate towards success.

They have your best interests at heart

Positive people are genuine, more so because they don't only care about themselves, but they care about you as well. It is important to them, as much as it is important to yourself, that you are feeling good about yourself or that your goals are met.

Influential

We tend to absorb the actions of those we spend a lot of time with. It is no doubt that by constantly being around these impactful and bright souls, you too will become a ray of sunshine!

Ways To Surround Yourself With Positive Energy

Have you ever entered someone's office or house and left feeling drained out. Do you find it difficult to talk to someone at a their personal spaces? Maybe there's a tension in the air or a stale odour that's bothering you; it could also be that someone in that space has been fighting and hurling hurtful words in the air; it could be anything so it's better to leave as soon as possible. Many times it's not the person, it's the atmosphere around you that might be contaminated with stressful energy

59. Keep Your Space Tidy And Clean

A neater desk results in more productive work than an untidy one. Always remember, your energy depends on your surroundings; so tidy up your comfortable spot and maintain it that way. Because good energy is blocked in chaotic and messy places. Ensure your cupboards and drawers are shut in your room before you go to bed, the bins should have a lid and avoid having too many accessories or furniture in black. Don't be a hoarder, you never know which old object might be having what energy, if you don't need it do away with it.

60. Practice Positive Thinking, Everyday And All The Time

Positive energy is stronger than negative and when you'll realise this, miracles will happen. It's easy to indulge in negative conversation when the other person starts it, but it's not worth all the bad karma that will eventually pollute the air and come back to you. if you find someone very grumpy, give them more love even if they don't deserve it. Sometimes the person who's the hardest to love needs it the most.

61. Sunshine Is The Best Medicine

Medical issues, mental health, the common stubborn cold or even to escape a particular person; step out and bask in all the golden rays of hope. There's a reason why it's called the 'Ray of hope'. Sunshine is indeed the most underrated natural therapy.

Instead Of Avoiding, Erase That Person Who Brings You Down From Your Life

We keep reading social media posts about driving that intoxicating friend of ours from New Year. But why do we always end up being at the receiving end while they remind us how inferior we are to the rest of the human race. Even though we feel bad for them and smilingly give them the last word but in order to be the bigger person we are carrying their negative energy with us. Tactfully step away if they don't succumb to your positivity.

62. Gratitude

The more you think about what you don't have the more chances there are you'll never get it. And if you don't thank the universe enough for what you have, you might lose that too. In simple words, grass is greener on the other side because it's probably fake. You're very lucky, just count your blessings.

63. Eat Good, Sleep Good, Read Good

The biggest truth that came with adulthood was the importance of sleep. Take out time for your sleep, nothing is more important. Eat good food because the sugar cravings are just giving you temporary happiness, it's not giving you good energy in the long run. You can only energise your body with enough sleep and enough wholesome food. And of course, self education makes you more aware of yourself and the world so keep reading to grow each day and attract the energy you want. It is a well known fact ' you are what you eat. We equally believe in the fact – you are what you read. Because that's what you think and attract.

64. Making Progress

Making progress can be linked to move forward in one's work or activity. Now this is how to know you are making progress in your relationship

How would you measure the progress of your relationship with the significant other? Some might view the level of understanding of each other's personality. Some might view the efforts spent on each other as an indication. Perhaps a few others would consider the monetary value of the gifts from the guy as a form of measurement? There are probably countless other ways. Personally, I would think that its very important to always assess if the relationship is progressing... whether there's a future together. And I would measure the progress and depth of a relationship in the following ways: There is mutual trust. Trust is arguably the key fundamental factor for the survival and growth of any relationship. However, building trust takes time and effort. It is slowly developed, honed and nurtured throughout the relationship. But it could also be shattered in a moment's folly. When you both have absolute confidence in each other's commitment towards the relationship, that's probably a damn good sign.

• No spying on and wiretapping each other's cell phones or calendars.

• No thoughts that your partner plans to run off with his/her attractive single friend.

You can probably feel it when there's that level of mutual trust present. It totally rocks doesn't it? Showing your real, true selves. In the initial stages of a relationship, some people (including myself) may put on certain 'fronts' for the other party, and hide some not-so-desirable characteristics of ourselves. Like peeling the numerous layers of an onion, you know when the relationship has progressed far when all the layers have been peeled and nothing is left but the true, innate self of that person. Transparent. Vulnerable. No more masks. No deception. Our deepest feelings and thoughts are shared with each other. We cry in front of each other. We talk about every single shit without holding back any secrets. Always encouraging each other. This is where the romantic Valentino would not be needed as it won't be about how excited you can make each other feel. Its time to be the best friend to your partner! To put on the hat of:

• Being a great confidante and listening to his/her problems.

• Being a great motivational coach and cheer him/her on.

And of course knowing the right words to say instead of making things worse (requires some experience). The best relationship is when you both can act as lovers and best friends at the same time. Ability to make each other laugh... always. The ability to make each other smile and laugh, ALWAYS, is probably a quality that comes only with a lot of mutual understanding and time spent together. Where all else in the world has failed to make you laugh – be it the humorous comedians or your favourite TV show Family Guy.

Only that partner of yours can do the trick. (well, maybe because he/she was the source of your unhappiness in the first place?) There are certain things that I can say to whoever I'm in love with to make he/she smile... all the time, whether they had a bad day or a good one. It's that magic 'laughter' formula that only you both know. It's about us, not just myself.

Some might say that love is selfish. Yeah its true if are participating in The Hunger Games to win the prize, which in this case is the person you like. But after you have weeded out the competition to win over the girl/guy, selflessness is probably a good indication about the depth of the relationship. It can no longer be about just your needs or pointing all faults at the other party. No longer can selfish opinions like this be held: "What's yours is now mine, but what's mine is still mine alone."

Accepting each other's flaws.

First of all, no one's perfect. Anyone who says they have no flaws ought to be shot. Anyone who says they need not work on their flaws ought to be flogged.

• It's easy to point to point out another's flaws no doubt. Anyone can do that.

• But in a great relationship, the couple can also accept each other's flaws, as well as acknowledge the flaws that our partners point out to us.

Personally, I know my relationship sorta progressed well when instead of merely pointing out the other person's mistakes, we both also started to admit our own flaws as well. (still Work-In-Progress though) Have patience with your partner's flaws, and the graciousness to admit your own.

Paying attention to small details.

The small details always matter. They are hardly noticeable at the infancy stage of a relationship but they should become more obvious to each party as the relationship progresses. Why? Simply because if a small details were overlooked, the potential effect could be HUGE and definitely NOTICEABLE. Yeah... you probably got that. Getting the wrong-coloured flowers may seem negligible from the perspective of guys, but it means a hell lot more to the girls. I know that... been there myself. The small details always matter.

Knowing how each other tick.

If a relationship has progressed far, there should probably be a good understanding of each other's 'love language', as coined by Gary Chapman in The 5 Love Languages.

• For instance, a guy feels that his own way of expressing love is through physical touch and does so to his girl.

• His girl however, prefers the love to be expressed through spending quality time together instead.

• This difference might cause the girl to think she is not loved sufficiently?

To avoid that, the guy should thus use the 'love language' that his partner would preferably like to receive. This takes a massive amount of time to figure out, man.

Leaving the past behind

A relationship cannot progress forward unless certain things are left behind. That includes past spats and disagreements about anything under the sun. It can be tiring and frustrating for a couple to constantly argue over the same old issues. Yeah... it is. Really. We are not archaeologists, so lets not dig up the past.

Seeing a future together.

After leaving the past behind, now is there a future ahead for us? I always ask myself these few questions:

• Do we have similar goals?

• Are our personalities compatible?

• Are we driven by the same things in life?

• Can I live with her on a daily basis?

It will probably be fuzzy and unclear in the earlier stages of the relationship, but the vision of the future should ideally become clearer as the relationship moves along. And if any differences can be ironed out, then I guess the relationship is getting somewhere great.

MINDSETS TO STAY AWAY FROM

Walking Around with Injured Looks

Human mind is a hub of activity. Depending on your interests, preoccupations and personality type, all sorts of thoughts can cross your mind; and there are thoughts that can give you an injured looking expression. Some such thoughts are: The boss doesn't recognize my merit; I am being underpaid; I am better than my co workers but paid less than them; I am deliberately not given the opportunity to excel; the boss probably doesn't like me. If you genuinely believe this to be true, talk to the management. Of course, be nice about it and don't ever make it sound personal by declaring nobody likes me. If nothing works, quit. And find some place where you think you can be more appreciated. However, if by chance you end up at such un-appreciative work places three times in a row, then most probably it is not chance. It's you. Try to work on your attitude. Remember, nothing is more off-putting than a person who thinks the entire world is conspiring to mistreat him/her.

Being Jealous of Your Co-Workers

Jealously almost always springs from low self esteem and lack of confidence. Some ways in which jealousy can manifest itself are: You find it difficult to like someone else's work; you can't bring yourself to celebrate a co-workers achievement; you find it downright torturous to compliment someone on a job well done. You may also harbor, conscious or unconscious, a jealously towards the boss. Surprisingly, this is quite common. Remember, a negative emotion like jealously is not only stressful but it also has a poisonous orbit. Your co-workers can sense it; your boss can feel it. People may not know why but they will feel uncomfortable in your company. But, like all other negative attitudes, jealousy is not something you are stuck with for good. You can always consciously work on being the best and most genuine version of you there could possibly be.

Passing the Buck

 Do you often point finger at others when you miss your deadlines? Do you often say 'It's not my fault, A was responsible for it'? If yes, you need to work on your tendency to blame others. Passing on the buck or holding others responsible for unfinished agendas and missed deadlines is an immature way to handle things and never sits well with the management. You will not only hamper your chances of success but will also fail to grow as an individual. One important mark of a well developed personality is the ability to take responsibility for your deadlines and act proactively instead of waiting for things to happen.

Taking Things Way Too Personally

Consider these scenarios: A co-worker makes a remark about your work and you believe the remark in some ways puts a dent on your authority. It's an official gathering, you are 10 minutes late and the co-workers start the party; for you, it's a trigger to dwell in that dark world where people have joined hands to undermine you. A co-worker didn't greet you, and you take it as a personal affront. You believe the co-worker deliberately ignored you.

Remember, the world doesn't revolve around you. People seldom make special arrangements to exclude you. People can forget; they can be preoccupied. And they probably don't even know you have a fragile ego that's easily riled.

Taking things personally is another sign that you are not comfortable in your own skin. Stop making comparisons, dwell on your positive attributes and try to acquire the skill-sets necessary for being successful in a job.

Not Being Able to Take Criticism

Criticism of your work or any facet of it could be simply what it seems on the surface: an opinion about or a remark on your work or some aspect of your work. Don't take it as a reflection on you as a person. If you constantly feel the need to be validated by other people, if any small criticism can impact your self-image in a big way, you are in the danger zone. Imagine living a life at the mercy of other peoples' opinions! Criticism, when taken in the right spirit, can go a long way in improving your work. It can offer new perspectives you may or may not have previously considered. Be open to criticism and try to see it for what it is: a point of view, an opinion from a different standpoint.

Remember, your worth as a person is not entirely dependent on the work you do. You are important in your own right as a unique human being that you are. Learn to let go of the need to find constant validation.

Treating your Job as a Time filler

You are treating your job as a time filler if your biggest aim in life is to somehow survive the 9-6 drudgery.

Okay, the job you are doing is not your true calling. You are putting up with the work you don't like because it helps you make a decent living. Or you are busy in learning what you actually want to do and decide to endure the ordeal till that happens. Don't. Nothing justifies such an attitude. No matter how much you try to camouflage it, this attitude will be reflected in the way you work, and the type of deliverables you make. Do aspire for higher things in life, but give your full attention to the work you are doing and while you are doing it. Loyalty and diligence are qualities that shine through no matter where you work. Besides, treating your job as a time filler is not just being dishonest it is also counterproductive. Life is not about filling empty hours. It is about living every moment and doing the things you can be proud of. Give the work you do your 120 percent, go an extra mile, be eager to accept responsibilities. Even a seemingly menial job when done with dedication and love can transform your outlook and can give you a sense of achievement so vital for living a satisfying life.

Ways to Measure Results in the Workplace

The modern workplace has changed drastically over the years. Gone are the days when employers only stressed the importance of results and profits. While it may still be a large part of assessing an employee's progress, today there are many things taken into consideration when measuring the productivity of workers. Today, results in the workplace exceed profits and results, and a company's reputation and how their workers assess them is also taken into consideration. How does the modern workplace measure results?

Team collaboration:

In addition to the finished product, companies are responsible for fostering an atmosphere that encourages teamwork and shared responsibility. If you're managing a project and are faced with a group of individuals that cannot get along and work together, the project could suffer immensely, deteriorating the results for the quarter. With increased teamwork and internal cohesiveness, team members will work together to solve problems and come up with creative solutions.

Social goal management:

One way to assess progress is to keep a track of employee goals on a regular basis. Having them set their personal short-term and long-term goals will allow the rest of the team to monitor their progress and make suggestions when necessary. Team members will be able to judge how well a project is going based on the work completed by others and can easily adjust project tasks accordingly.

Employee satisfaction:

Discontent employees means loss of productivity at work. Similiar to team collaboration, workers appreciate healthy office environments and having the chance to collaborate and be rewarded for a job well done. The more satisfied workers are with their projects, co-workers and bosses, the harder they will work to achieve their goals and make an impact within the organization.

CONCLUSION

Thank you for reading this book. It is my hope that I have managed to make a small difference to your lifestyle by offering you some great suggestions on how to improve the quality of your life. From this point on, it is up to you, my dear reader to choose which habits you will try and which don't. The only thing I want you to keep in mind is that every small habit has a massive impact if practiced on a regular basis. If you can't see the difference every day, it doesn't mean that nothing is happening. Small changes are easy to ake and have a " compound interest " effect on your life but it takes time to see the change.

As as ancient French proverb sais, "Rome ne s'est pas faite en un jour. (Rome wasn't built in a day.)"

If you have enjoyed this book, check out my other books in the same series.